# PRE DIABETES COOKBOOK

Delicious Recipes To Keep You Healthy And Lower Your Blood Sugar

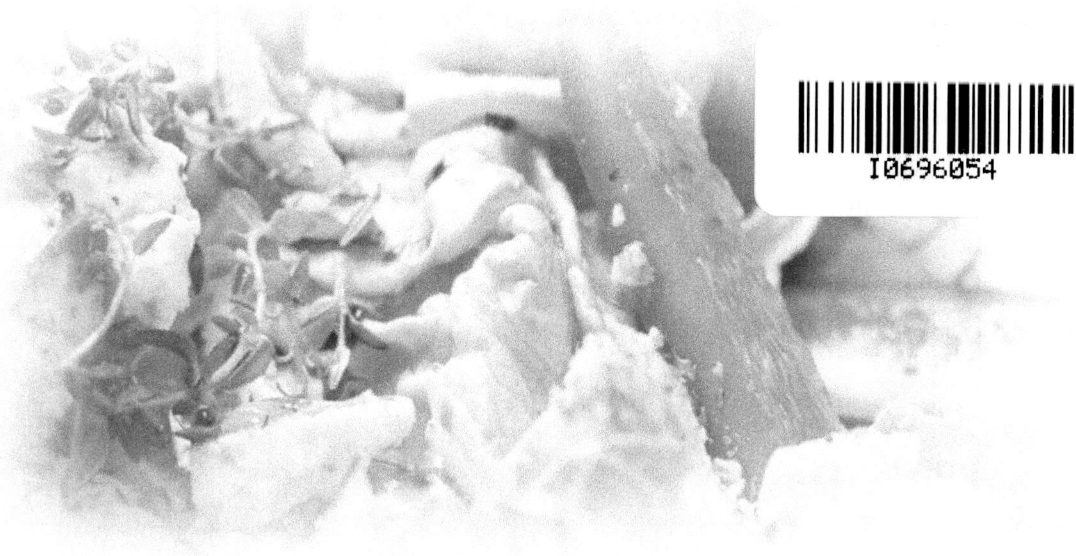

DOROTHY BEATRICE

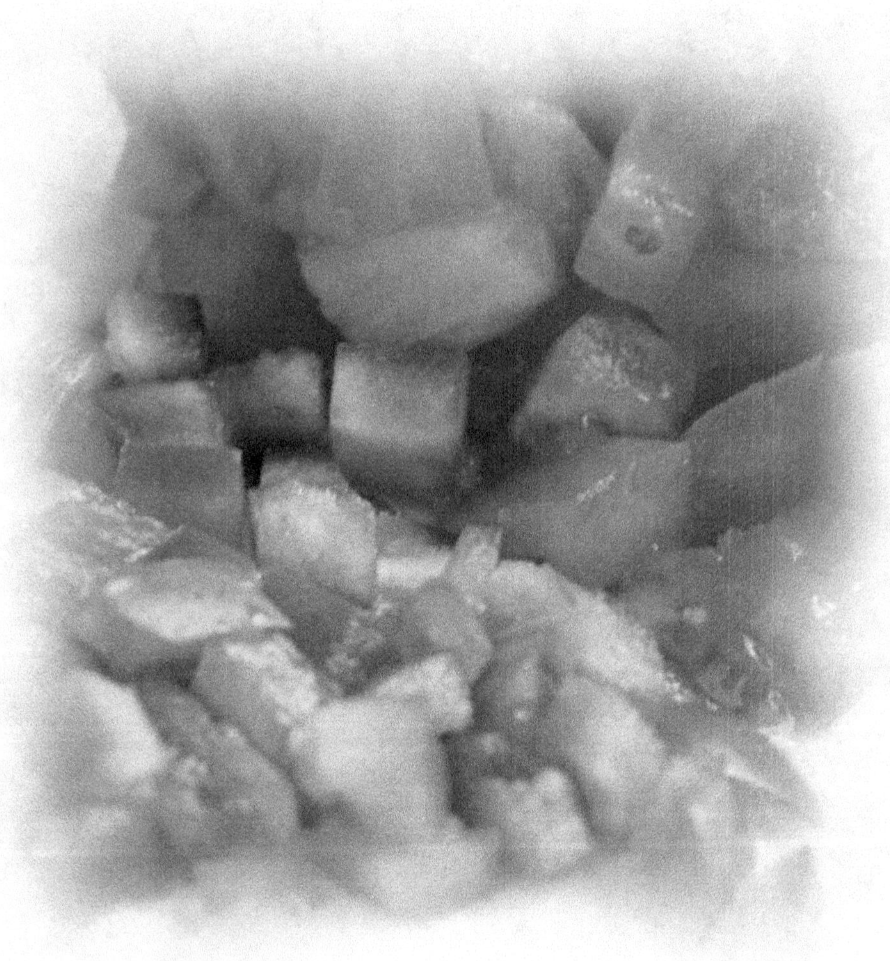

# INTRODUCTION

If you're reading this cookbook, you undoubtedly have some pre-diabetes-related questions or concerns. You're not alone, so don't worry. I pledge to make things fun, straightforward, and idea-filled as we embark on this adventure together.

Okay, let's first clarify the facts. Pre-diabetes is comparable to a flashing yellow light. It's the universe's way of telling you to take it easy and assess your wellbeing. Although your blood sugar is higher than normal, it is not yet diabetes. It serves as a heads-up and an alert.

Think of your body as a vehicle. If gasoline is its fuel, then blood sugar (also known as glucose) is much like the oil. We require it to maintain order, but too much or too little can lead to issues.

Probably you've heard the saying "You are what you eat." Though it may sound corny, it's actually extremely true. Particularly when discussing blood sugar. In this battle against pre-diabetes, your diet can either be your best friend or deadliest enemy.

Consider your preferred dish. Yummy, yes? Currently, certain foods cause our blood sugar levels to soar then plummet, like a rollercoaster. However, who enjoys the frightful fall on roller coasters? We want a smooth, enjoyable ride. And this cookbook fills that need! We'll locate meals that will provide you a comfortable, enjoyable ride while controlling your blood sugar.

You may be asking, "How can this book help me?" at this point. wonderful question

First, I've assembled a ton of delectable dishes (since who said nutritious food needs to be bland?). These dishes are designed to keep your blood sugar constant while yet tasting tasty.

Imagine having a helpful neighbor who occasionally drops by to chat; that's me, but in book form!

Finally, we'll debunk several myths around pre-diabetes. You'll feel knowledgeable, in control, and perhaps even a little peckish by the time you're done (but don't worry, we've got the recipes covered). It will be a pleasant journcy, I promise.

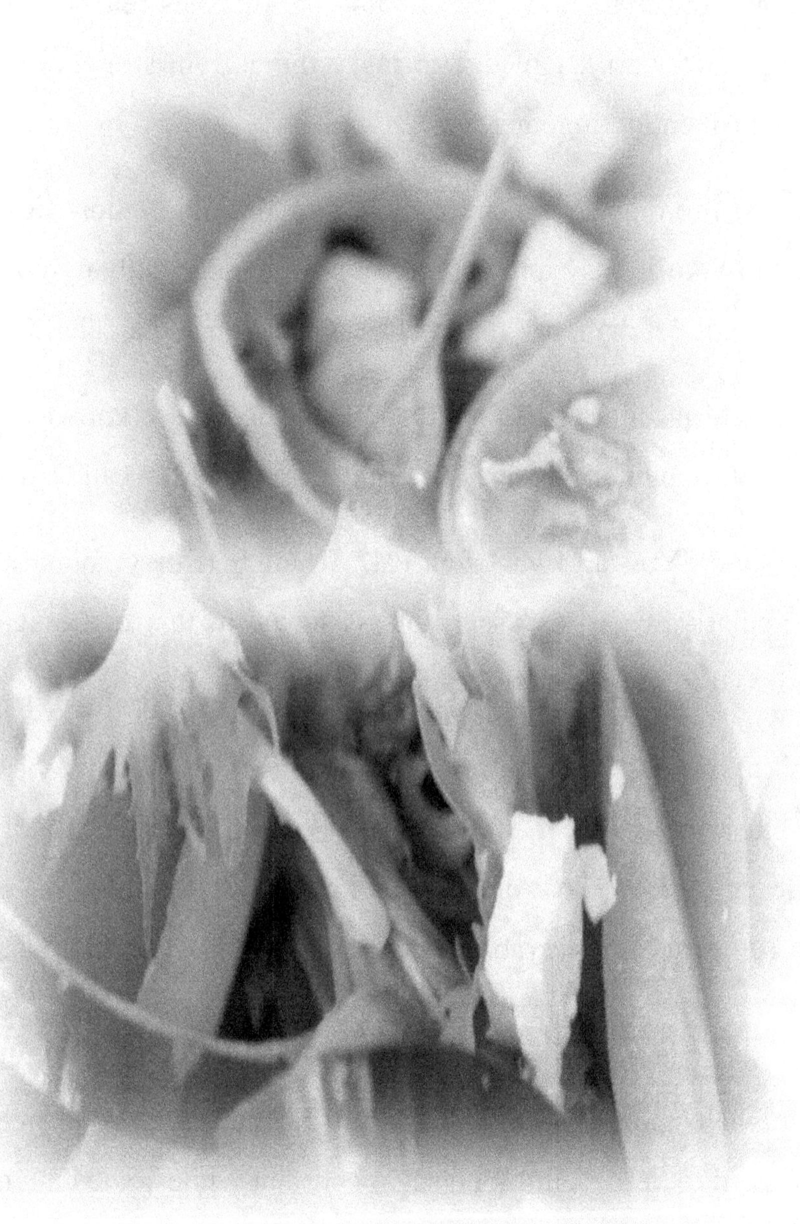

# CHAPTER 1

# THE PRE-DIABETES SCIENCE

Think of the energy system in your body as a busy metropolis. This city's inhabitants are your cells, and they require energy to keep things operating properly. Our main source of energy? glucose, a sugar found in food.

Glucose requires a key to enter the cells in order to be functional. Insulin is the key, and the pancreas makes it. But occasionally, our cells develop an insulin resistance. They resemble irate landlords who secretly changed the locks on their apartments. In response, the pancreas produces more insulin to facilitate glucose uptake by cells. However, it can have trouble keeping up over time. The outcome? Pre-diabetes is a condition marked by elevated blood sugar levels.

## Why Should You Give Pre-Diabetes Any Attention?

Pre-diabetes is a warning, like a yellow traffic signal. Although it's not a guarantee, it's a definite indication you're headed down the path to type 2 diabetes. Additionally, it is important to pay attention to this warning sign because diabetes is associated with a wide range of health issues, such as kidney damage, heart disease, and stroke.

## Symptoms of pre diabetes

Pre-diabetes typically has very mild or no symptoms. Blood testing are the most reliable approach to determine for certain. The most typical exams are:

Fasting Blood Glucose Test: If your blood sugar level is between 100 and 125 mg/dl after an overnight fast, you are pre-diabetic.

Hemoglobin A1c test: This gauges your average blood sugar level over a period of two to three months. When the result ranges from 5.7% to 6.4%, pre-diabetes is present.

Don't freak out if either of these tests finds you to be pre-diabetic. Consider it as a step in the direction of a healthy way of life.

## Diabetes Resistance

Ever nod along while seeming to understand when someone uses the word "insulin resistance" in a sentence? I'm not passing judgment; we've all been there. However, let's examine it today so that you can confidently nod the next time.



Let's review what should occur before we get into what goes wrong with insulin resistance. Consider insulin to be a crucial. Following a meal, our body converts the food into glucose, a form of sugar, which is then absorbed into the bloodstream. For glucose to give our cells energy, it must enter the cells. The pancreas's production of insulin fills this need. It works as a key to open up cells so that glucose can get inside. All is well thus far, right?

## Resistantance

Imagine that our cells' locks eventually become rusted or difficult to operate. It gets more difficult to unlock the door even with the correct key (insulin). Insulin resistance appears in this circumstance. Because the body's cells don't react to insulin as well, glucose has a difficult time entering.

The pancreas responds by producing more insulin, thinking, "No problem, I'll just make more keys!". The pancreas may eventually become exhausted and be unable to produce adequate insulin. The outcome? rising amounts of blood sugar.

Insulin resistance is comparable to a covert leak in your home. You might not notice it at first, but if you ignore it, it could develop into a bigger issue. Type 2 diabetes may be facilitated by persistently increased blood sugar levels. Also not ideal are excessive insulin levels, which have been related to a variety of problems including obesity, heart disease, and more.



Genetics: You may be more vulnerable if your mother, father, or grandmother had type 2 diabetes or insulin resistance. A family affair, that is.

Weight: Excess weight, especially around the abdomen, can increase the insulin resistance of cells.

Muscles don't consume as much glucose when people lead sedentary lifestyles, which causes a buildup in the blood.

unsound diet Frequent fast food binges and sugary indulgences are bad for our insulin response. Other aspects Certain medical conditions, including polycystic ovarian syndrome (PCOS), drugs, and even sleep issues may contribute.

## Signs and Symptoms of Insulin Resistance

Insulin resistance may operate covertly. Most people don't realize they have it until they are given a type 2 diabetes diagnosis. However, some indicators could alert you:

**Darkened Skin Patches:** A condition known as acanthosis nigricans may appear on the neck or beneath the arms.

Being regularly exhausted, even after a restful night's sleep, can be an indication.

**Cravings:** More than just a sweet tooth acting up, an unquenchable craving for carbohydrates and sugars may signal a problem.

Please bear with me if you think this whole thing sounds depressing. The good news? In order to treat insulin resistance, you can:

**Exercise:** Exercise reduces the amount of insulin needed by cells to utilise glucose. A little stroll, a dance lesson, or a bike ride can have an impact.

**Eat Wisely**: Give foods that regulate blood sugar top priority. Your allies should be whole grains, vegetables, lean proteins, and healthy fats. Furthermore, choosing water over sugary beverages is a game-changer.

Loss of weight Reduced body weight can enhance insulin sensitivity even slightly. Progress rather than perfection is the goal.

**Sleep Well:** Everyone benefits from a restful night's sleep. Regular, sound sleep aids in the control of insulin and blood sugar.

**Control Stress:** It's true that saying than doing. However, methods like meditation, deep breathing, and even interests can assist manage stress.

## Why Glycemic Index Is Important

Think about being at a party. Some visitors show up and immediately get involved (imagine them as the party's life), while others take their time and mingle slowly. Similar concepts underlie the Glycemic Index (GI), but for carbohydrates. It gauges how rapidly a food high in carbohydrates elevates blood sugar levels after consumption.

Foods are rated by GI on a scale of 0 to 100:

The "life of the party" carbohydrates are those with a high GI (70 and higher). They cause a sharp blood sugar increase. Examples? White bread, potatoes, and a variety of morning cereals.

The guests with a medium GI (56 to 69) fall into this category. They gradually elevate blood sugar levels. Consider honey, whole wheat goods, and some fruits, such as pineapples.

Low GI (55 or less): Your relaxed, softly mingling carbohydrates. They gradually affect blood sugar. Most veggies, beans, and lentils fall within this category.

**Here is why the GI is important:**

Energy Security Foods with a low GI provide longer-lasting energy. No more crashing after a sugar rush!

**Hunger & Weight Control:** Low-GI foods can keep you satiated for longer, helping with weight management.

**For diabetics:** Diabetes patients must carefully control their blood sugar levels. Their toolset may contain a good understanding of GI.

**Heart Wellness:** According to some research, a low-GI diet can lower cholesterol levels, which is good for heart health.

**Glycemic Load (GL):** This factor considers both the food's GI and its carbohydrate content. A food may occasionally have a high GI but a low GL because it has few carbohydrates. A well-known example is watermelon.

nutritive worth: Not all low-GI foods are excellent sources of nourishment. conversely as well! The GI of some nutrient-dense foods may be greater. It's crucial to take the total nutritional package into account.

Here are some tips if you're considering incorporating the Glycemic Index into your daily life:

**Balance It Out:** Aim for a balanced dish rather than concentrating primarily on GI. Combine carbohydrates with protein, good fats, and a lot of vegetables.

**Healthy Eating First:** Give whole, unprocessed foods a priority. Many are naturally lower in GI and are rich in vital nutrients.

**Keep an Open Mind When Reading Labels:** Even while some items claim to have a low GI, they may be packed with unwholesome components. Always consider the bigger picture of nutrition.

**Take Note of Your Body:** The way each person's body responds varies. Some people may thrive on low-GI meals, while others may require a combination. Pay attention to how some certain foods make you feel.

**Go for Variety:** It involves more than just eating only low-GI foods. By varying your dietary selections, you may make sure you're getting a variety of nutrients.

Prioritize These Foods for Blood Sugar Health

All of the cells in our bodies receive their energy from blood sugar, also known as blood glucose, which is the sugar that is delivered in our bloodstream. Imagine it as a VIP guest at the energy celebration that our cells throw. Things go smoothly when it is at the ideal level. If it's too high or too low, though? Well, there might be a few health issues that show up and ruin the party.

## Important Foods to Balance Blood Sugar

Blood sugar control is comparable to perfecting the tightrope walking technique. It's a fine line to walk! Fortunately, several nutrients take center stage in this delicate balancing act:

**Fiber**: Fiber delays the absorption of sugar, causing blood sugar levels to rise more gradually.

Where can you get it? The more leafy the vegetable, the better, the fruit (apples with the skin on, berries), the legume (beans, lentils), and the nuts & seeds (chia seeds, flaxseeds).

**Chromium:** It improves the function of insulin, the hormone in charge of allowing sugar to enter our cells.

Where can you get it? Green beans, broccoli, nutritious grains, and almonds.

Increasing insulin sensitivity may be aided by omega-3 fatty acids.

Where can you get it? chia seeds, walnuts, flaxseeds, and fatty fish like salmon.

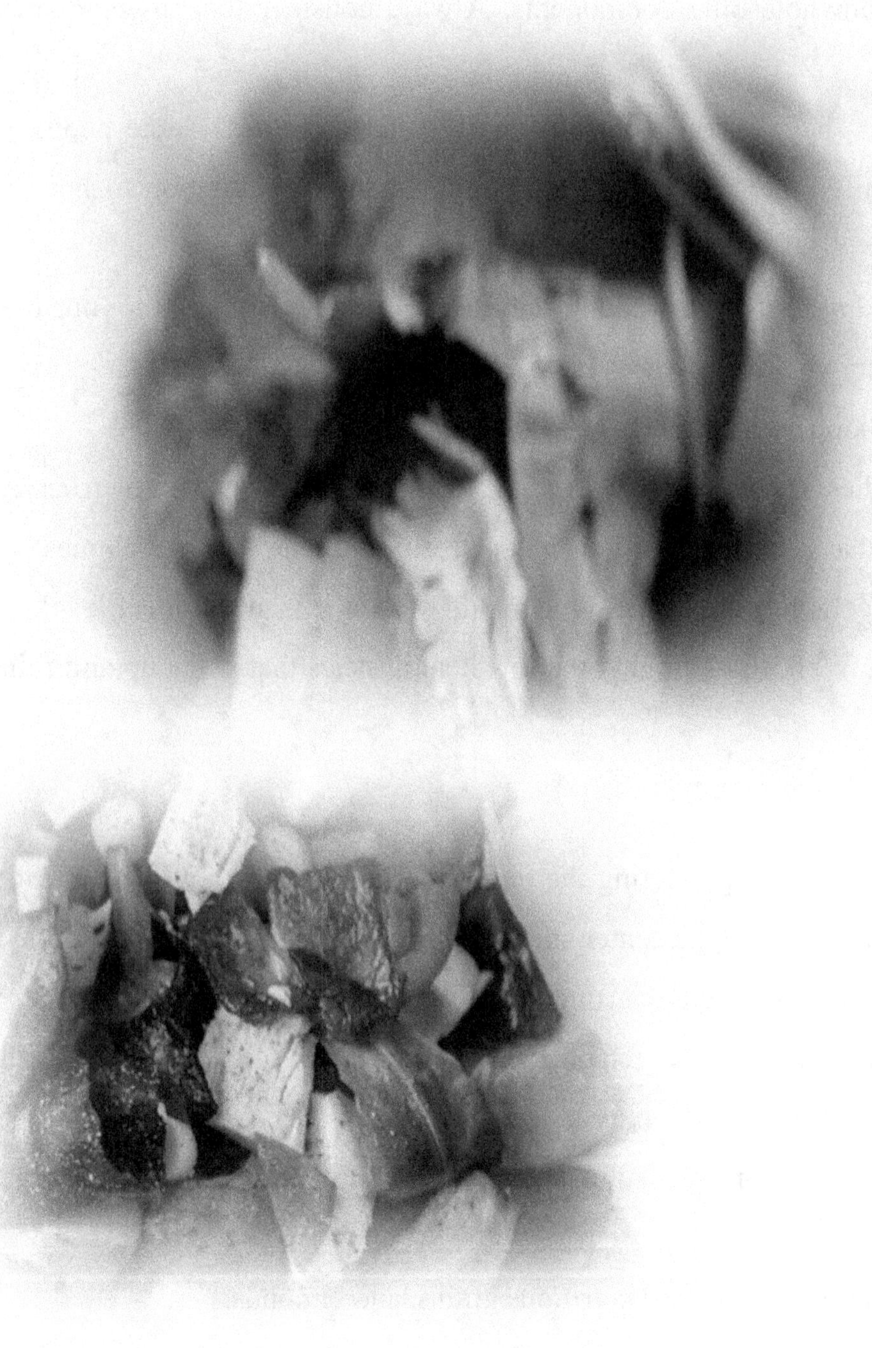

## Chia Seed Pudding

Prep Time: 10 minutes (+ overnight soaking)

Servings: 2

**Ingredients:**

4 tbsp chia seeds

2 cups unsweetened almond milk

1 tsp vanilla extract

1 tbsp maple syrup or stevia

Fresh fruit for topping (e.g., berries)

**Preparation Method:**

Combine chia seeds, almond milk, vanilla extract, and maple syrup or stevia in a mixing dish.

Stir thoroughly to avoid clumping.

Refrigerate overnight, covered.

Give it a thorough swirl before serving and garnish with fresh fruit.

Nutritional Information (approx per serving):

Calories: 190

Carbs: 20g

Protein: 5g

Fat: 10g

Fiber: 8g



## Avocado & Egg on Whole Grain Toast

Prep Time: 10 minutes

Servings: 1

**Ingredients:**

1 slice whole grain toast

½ ripe avocado

1 large egg

Salt & pepper to taste

Pinch of chili flakes (optional)

**Preparation Method:**

Toast the whole grain bread until it reaches the desired crispiness.

Spread the avocado mash on the toast.

Cook the egg to your liking (fried or poached) on a nonstick pan.

On top of the avocado spread, place the egg.

Season with salt, pepper, and chili powder to taste.

Nutritional Information (approx):

Calories: 300

Carbs: 20g

Protein: 12g

Fat: 20g

Fiber: 7g

## Veggie Omelette

Prep Time: 15 minutes

Servings: 1

**Ingredients:**

2 large eggs

¼ cup bell peppers, diced

¼ cup mushrooms, sliced

¼ cup spinach, chopped

1 tbsp olive oil

Salt & pepper to taste

**Preparation Method:**

Combine the eggs, salt, and pepper and mix in a bowl.

In a nonstick skillet, heat the olive oil.

Cook until the bell peppers and mushrooms are softened.

Cook until the spinach has wilted.

Pour in the beaten eggs, making sure the vegetables are well distributed.

Cook until the center is firm, then flip and cook the other side.

Nutritional Information (approx):

Calories: 250

Carbs: 5g

Protein: 14g

Fat: 19g

Fiber: 2g

## Greek Yogurt with Nuts & Berries

Prep Time: 5 minutes

Servings: 1

**Ingredients:**

1 cup Greek yogurt (unsweetened)

¼ cup mixed berries (blueberries, raspberries, etc.)

¼ cup mixed nuts (almonds, walnuts, etc.)

1 tsp honey (optional)

**Preparation Method:**

In a dish, combine Greek yogurt, berries, and mixed nuts. Drizzle with honey, if preferred.

Nutritional Information (approx):

Calories: 280

Carbs: 20g

Protein: 20g

Fat: 15g

Fiber: 3g

## Steel-Cut Oats with Almonds & Blueberries

Prep Time: 25 minutes

Servings: 2

**Ingredients:**

1 cup steel-cut oats

2.5 cups water

¼ cup blueberries

¼ cup sliced almonds

1 tbsp maple syrup or stevia

**Preparation Method:**

Boil water in a pot

Reduce the heat to a simmer and add the steel-cut oats.

Cook, stirring periodically, for 20-25 minutes, or until the oats are soft.

Top with blueberries and almonds in individual dishes.

Drizzle with maple syrup or stevia to taste.

Nutritional Information (approx per serving):

Calories: 250

Carbs: 35g

Protein: 8g

Fat: 9g

Fiber: 5g

## Low-Carb Smoothie

Prep Time: 5 minutes

Servings: 1

**Ingredients:**

1 cup unsweetened almond milk

½ avocado

¼ cup raspberries

1 tbsp chia seeds

1 scoop protein powder (optional)

Ice cubes

**Preparation Method:**

In a blender, combine all of the ingredients.

Blend until completely smooth.

Nutritional Information (approx):

Calories: 220

Carbs: 12g

Protein: 8g (more if protein powder added)

Fat: 16g

Fiber: 8g

## Cottage Cheese & Fruit Bowl

Prep Time: 5 minutes

Servings: 1

**Ingredients:**

1 cup low-fat cottage cheese

¼ cup mixed fruit (berries, kiwi, etc.)

1 tbsp sunflower seeds

1 tsp honey (optional)

**Preparation Method:**

In a bowl, combine the cottage cheese.

Serve with fresh fruit and sunflower seeds on top.

If desired, drizzle with honey.

Nutritional Information (approx):

Calories: 210

Carbs: 15g

Protein: 25g

Fat: 5g

Fiber: 2g

## Quinoa & Veggie Stir Fry

Prep Time: 20 minutes

Servings: 2

**Ingredients:**

1 cup cooked quinoa

1 cup mixed veggies (bell peppers, broccoli, zucchini, etc.)

1 tbsp olive oil

1 clove garlic, minced

1 tbsp low-sodium soy sauce

Salt & pepper to taste

**Preparation Method:**

Put the olive oil and heat in a pan.

Garlic should be sautéed until aromatic.

Stir in the mixed vegetables until they are tender crisp.

Add the cooked quinoa, soy sauce, salt, and pepper to taste.

Cook for another 2-3 minutes, stirring often.

Nutritional Information (approx per serving):

Calories: 250

Carbs: 35g

Protein: 8g

Fat: 9g

Fiber: 5g

## Whole Grain Pancakes with Almond Butter

Prep Time: 20 minutes

Servings: 2

**Ingredients:**

1 cup whole grain pancake mix

1 cup water (or as per mix instructions)

2 tbsp almond butter

Fresh fruit for topping (optional)

Maple syrup or stevia for drizzling (optional)

**Preparation Method:**

Make the pancake batter according to the package instructions.

Put a nonstick skillet or griddle over medium heat.

Pour the batter into the pan. Cook until bubbles appear on the surface, then turn and cook the other side.

Serve with almond butter, fresh fruit, and, if desired, a drizzle of syrup or stevia.

Nutritional Information (approx per serving):

Calories: 320

Carbs: 45g

Protein: 9g

Fat: 12g

Fiber: 6g

## Tofu Scramble

Prep Time: 15 minutes

Servings: 2

**Ingredients:**

1 cup firm tofu, crumbled

¼ cup bell peppers, diced

¼ cup tomatoes, diced

¼ cup onions, chopped

1 tbsp olive oil

½ tsp turmeric

Salt & pepper to taste

**Preparation Method:**

Put the olive oil in a nonstick skillet and heat.

Cook until the onions are transparent.

Cook for a few minutes after adding the bell peppers and tomatoes.

Toss in the crushed tofu, turmeric, salt, and pepper.

Cook for 5-7 minutes.

Nutritional Information (approx per serving):

Calories: 180

Carbs: 8g

Protein: 12g

Fat: 12g

Fiber: 3g

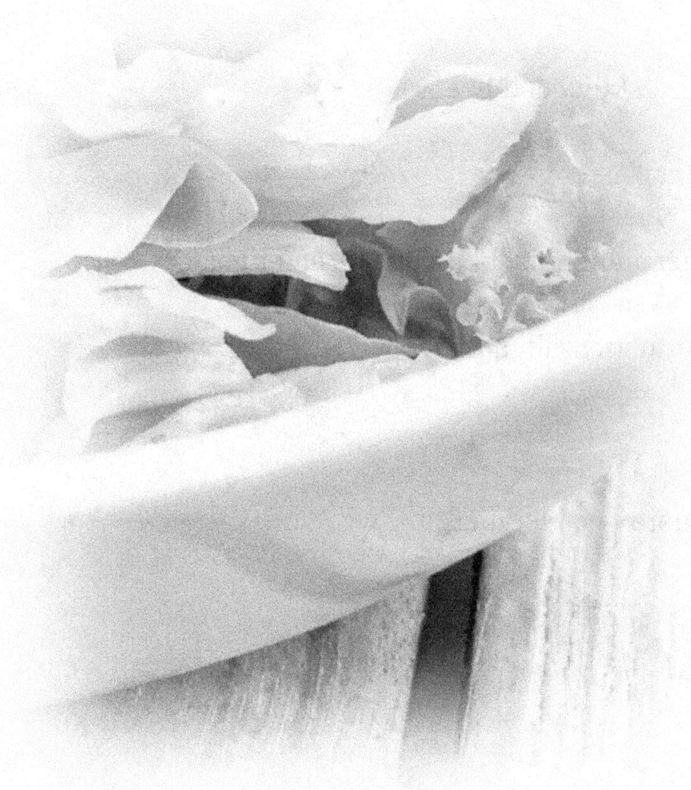

### Grilled Chicken Salad

Prep Time: 15 minutes

Cook Time: 15 minutes

Servings: 4

**Ingredients:**

4 boneless, skinless chicken breasts

8 cups mixed salad greens

1 cup cherry tomatoes, halved

1 cucumber, sliced

¼ cup feta cheese, crumbled (optional)

2 tablespoons olive oil

2 tablespoons balsamic vinegar

Salt and pepper to taste

**Preparation Method:**

Preheat the grill on medium heat.

Salt and pepper the chicken breasts.

Grill the chicken for 6-7 minutes on each side, or until done.

Salad greens, cherry tomatoes, and cucumber should all be combined in a large mixing dish.

Add grilled chicken slices to the salad.

Sprinkle with olive oil, balsamic vinegar, and, if preferred, feta cheese. Toss thoroughly before serving.

Nutritional Information (per serving):

Calories: 230

Carbohydrates: 5g

Protein: 28g

Fat: 10g

Fiber: 2g

Sugars: 3g

## Vegetable Lentil Soup

Prep Time: 15 minutes

Cook Time: 45 minutes

Servings: 6

**Ingredients:**

1 cup green lentils, rinsed

2 tablespoons olive oil

1 onion, diced

2 carrots, diced

2 celery stalks, diced

2 cloves garlic, minced

8 cups vegetable broth

1 bay leaf

1 teaspoon dried thyme

2 cups kale or spinach, chopped

Salt and pepper to taste

**Preparation Method:**

Heat olive oil in a large pot. Sauté the onion, carrots, and celery until tender.

Cook for another 1-2 minutes after adding the garlic.

Combine the vegetable broth, lentils, bay leaf, and thyme in a mixing bowl. Bring the water to a boil.

Reduce the heat to low and cook for 30 minutes, or until the lentils are soft.

Cook for another 5 minutes after adding the kale or spinach.

Season with salt and pepper to taste. Before serving, remove the bay leaf.

Nutritional Information (per serving):

Calories: 190

Carbohydrates: 30g

Protein: 10g

Fat: 4g

Fiber: 12g

Sugars: 4g

## Quinoa and Black Bean Bowl

Prep Time: 20 minutes

Cook Time: 25 minutes

Servings: 4

**Ingredients:**

1 cup quinoa

2 cups water

15 oz black beans, rinsed and drained

1 red bell pepper, diced

1 cup corn kernels

2 green onions, chopped

¼ cup fresh cilantro, chopped

2 tablespoons olive oil

1 tablespoon lime juice

Salt and pepper to taste

**Preparation Method:**

Boil water in a potCover and adjust heat to low.  Cook  until the quinoa is tender.

Combine cooked quinoa, black beans, bell pepper, corn, green onions, and cilantro in a large mixing dish.

In a separate bowl, combine the olive oil, lime juice, salt, and pepper.  Toss the quinoa mixture with the dressing to mix properly.

Nutritional Information (per serving):

Calories: 310

Carbohydrates: 50g

Protein: 12g

Fat: 8g

Fiber: 8g

Sugars: 4g

## Stuffed Bell Peppers

Prep Time: 20 minutes

Cook Time: 40 minutes

Servings: 4

**Ingredients:**

4 large bell peppers (any color)

1 lb lean ground turkey or chicken

1 cup cooked brown rice

1 can (14 oz) diced tomatoes, drained

1 onion, fincly chopped

2 cloves garlic, minced

1 tsp ground cumin

Salt and pepper to taste

1 cup shredded low-fat cheddar cheese (optional)

**Preparation Method:**

Preheat the oven to 375 degrees Fahrenheit.

Remove the seeds from the bell peppers and Place aside.

Cook ground turkey, onion, and garlic in a skillet until turkey is browned.

Add rice, tomatoes, cumin, salt, and pepper to taste.

Fill each bell pepper halfway with the turkey-rice mixture.

Cover the peppers in a baking dish with foil.

Put in the oven 35 minutes. If using cheese, sprinkle on top and bake for 5 minutes more, or until melted.

Nutritional Information (per serving):

Calories: 280

Carbohydrates: 30g

Protein: 25g

Fat: 7g

Fiber: 5g

Sugars: 6g

**Spinach and Feta Stuffed Chicken Breast**

Prep Time: 20 minutes

Cook Time: 25 minutes

Servings: 4

**Ingredients:**

4 boneless, skinless chicken breasts

2 cups fresh spinach, chopped

½ cup feta cheese, crumbled

1 tsp olive oil

2 cloves garlic, minced

Salt and pepper to taste

**Preparation Method:**

Preheat the oven to 375 degrees Fahrenheit.

Heat olive oil in a skillet and sauté garlic until the scent comes out.Cook until the spinach has wilted.

Remove from the fire and stir in the feta cheese. Season with salt and pepper to taste.

Each chicken breast should be stuff with the spinach-feta mixture.

In a baking dish, place the chicken breasts. Season with salt and pepper to taste.

Bake for 20-25 minutes, or until the chicken is thoroughly done.

Nutritional Information (per serving):

Calories: 210

Carbohydrates: 2g

Protein: 30g

Fat: 8g

Fiber: 0.5g

Sugars: 1g

## Broccoli and Cauliflower Stir-Fry

Prep Time: 15 minutes

Cook Time: 10 minutes

Servings: 4

**Ingredients:**

2 cups broccoli florets

2 cups cauliflower florets

1 bell pepper, sliced

2 tbsp olive oil

2 tbsp low-sodium soy sauce

1 tsp sesame oil

2 cloves garlic, minced

1 tbsp ginger, minced

**Preparation Method:**

In a wok or big skillet, heat the olive oil over medium-high heat.

Sauté the garlic and ginger for a minute, or until fragrant.

Combine the broccoli, cauliflower, and bell pepper. Cook  until the vegetables are soft.

Drizzle with sesame oil and soy sauce. To blend, stir everything together thoroughly.

Nutritional Information (per serving):

Calories: 110

Carbohydrates: 10g

Protein: 3g

Fat: 7g

Fiber: 3g

Sugars: 3g

## Chickpea and Vegetable Curry

Prep Time: 15 minutes

Cook Time: 30 minutes

Servings: 6

**Ingredients:**

1 can (14 oz) chickpeas, rinsed and drained

2 cups diced tomatoes

1 onion, chopped

2 cloves garlic, minced

1 tbsp curry powder

½ cup light coconut milk

2 cups mixed vegetables (e.g. peas, carrots, bell peppers)

1 tbsp olive oil

Salt and pepper to taste

**Preparation Method:**

The olive oil should be heated in a large skillet.

Cook until the onion and garlic are softened.

Cook for another minute after adding the curry powder.

Combine the tomatoes, chickpeas, mixed veggies, and coconut milk in a mixing bowl.

Cook for 25-30 minutes, or until the veggies are soft and the flavors have melded.

Season with salt and pepper.

Nutritional Information (per serving):

Calories: 180

Carbohydrates: 28g

Protein: 6g

Fat: 5g

Fiber: 7g

Sugars: 6g

## Zucchini Noodles with Pesto and Cherry Tomatoes

Prep Time: 15 minutes

Cook Time: 5 minutes

Servings: 4

**Ingredients:**

4 medium zucchinis, spiralized into noodles

1 cup cherry tomatoes, halved

½ cup pesto (store-bought or homemade with olive oil, basil, garlic, pine nuts, and parmesan)

2 tbsp olive oil

Salt and pepper to taste

Grated Parmesan for garnish (optional)

**Preparation Method:**

The olive oil should be heated in a large skillet.

Sauté the zucchini noodles until slightly softened.

Combine the cherry tomatoes and pesto in a mixing bowl. To mix, toss everything together.

Season with salt and pepper to taste. Cook for another 2 minutes.

If preferred, top with grated Parmesan cheese.

Nutritional Information (per serving):

Calories: 190

Carbohydrates: 10g

Protein: 5g

Fat: 15g

Fiber: 3g

Sugars: 5g

## Grilled Salmon with Steamed Asparagus

Prep Time: 10 minutes

Cook Time: 15 minutes

Servings: 4

**Ingredients:**

4 salmon fillets (5-6 oz each)

1 bunch of asparagus, trimmed

2 tbsp olive oil

2 cloves garlic, minced

Lemon zest and juice of 1 lemon

Salt and pepper to taste

**Preparation Method:**

Preheat the grill to medium-high.

Salmon fillets should be rubbed with olive oil, lemon zest, garlic, salt, and pepper.

Grill the salmon for 5-6 minutes on each side, or until cooked through.

Meanwhile, steam the asparagus for 4-5 minutes, or until tender-crisp.

Sprinkle lemon juice over asparagus and season with salt and pepper.

Serve the salmon with steamed asparagus as a side dish.

Nutritional Information (per serving):

Calories: 260

Carbohydrates: 5g

Protein: 30g

Fat: 13g

Fiber: 2g

Sugars: 2g

## Eggplant and Mushroom Ratatouille

Prep Time: 20 minutes

Cook Time: 40 minutes

Servings: 6

**Ingredients:**

1 large eggplant, diced

2 cups mushrooms, sliced

1 onion, chopped

1 bell pepper, diced

2 zucchinis, diced

1 can (14 oz) diced tomatoes

2 cloves garlic, minced

2 tbsp olive oil

1 tsp dried basil

1 tsp dried oregano

Salt and pepper to taste

**Preparation Method:**

The olive oil should be heated in a large skillet.

Sauté the onion and garlic until tender.

Combine the eggplant, mushrooms, bell peppers, and zucchinis in a mixing bowl. Cook  until the vegetables soften.

Toss in the diced tomatoes, basil, oregano, salt, and pepper to taste. Combine thoroughly.

Reduce the heat to low, cover, and cook for 25-30 minutes, or until all of the veggies are soft and the flavors have melded.

 Taste and adjust the seasonings.

Nutritional Information (per serving):

Calories: 120

Carbohydrates: 20g

Protein: 4g

Fat: 5g

Fiber: 6g

Sugars: 8g

### Baked Lemon Herb Salmon

Prep Time: 10 minutes

Cook Time: 20 minutes

Servings: 4

**Ingredients:**

4 salmon fillets

2 tablespoons olive oil

1 lemon (sliced)

2 cloves garlic (minced)

2 tablespoons fresh dill (chopped)

Salt and pepper to taste

**Preparation Method:**

Preheat the oven to 375 degrees Fahrenheit.

Salmon fillets should be placed in a baking dish.

In a mixing bowl, combine the olive oil, minced garlic, dill, salt, and pepper.

Drizzle the salmon fillets with the mixture.

Lemon slices should be put on top of each fillet.

Bake the salmon for 20 minutes.

Nutritional Information (per serving):

Calories: 230

Carbs: 1g

 Protein: 25g

Fat: 14g

Fiber: 0.5g

Sugar: 0g

## Stir-Fried Tofu with Vegetables

Prep Time: 15 minutes

Cook Time: 15 minutes

Servings: 4

**Ingredients:**

1 block firm tofu (cubed)

2 cups broccoli florets

1 bell pepper (sliced)

1 carrot (sliced)

2 tablespoons soy sauce (low sodium)

2 tablespoons olive oil

2 cloves garlic (minced)

1 tablespoon ginger (grated)

1 tablespoon sesame seeds

**Preparation Method:**

 Heat the olive oil in a skillet.

Sauté the garlic and ginger until fragrant.

Fry the tofu cubes till golden brown.

Stir-fry the vegetables for around 5 minutes.

Toss in the soy sauce to coat evenly.

Serve garnished with sesame seeds.

Nutritional Information (per serving):

Calories: 210

Carbs: 10g

Protein: 12g

Fat: 14g

Fiber: 3g

Sugar: 4g

## Grilled Vegetable Platter

Prep Time: 15 minutes

Cook Time: 10 minutes

Servings: 4

**Ingredients:**

1 zucchini (sliced)

1 bell pepper (quartered)

1 red onion (sliced)

8 cherry tomatoes

2 tablespoons olive oil

Salt and pepper to taste

2 tablespoons balsamic vinegar

**Preparation Method:**

Preheat the grill to medium-high.

Toss the veggies with the olive oil, salt, and pepper to taste.

Grill the vegetables for about 5 minutes on each side, or until they have grill marks.

Remove from the grill and serve drizzled with balsamic vinegar.

Nutritional Information (per serving):

Calories: 100

Carbs: 10g

Protein: 2g

Fat: 7g

Fiber: 2g

Sugar: 6g

Spaghetti Squash with Marinara Sauce

Prep Time: 10 minutes

Cook Time: 40 minutes

Servings: 4

**Ingredients:**

1 spaghetti squash (halved and seeds removed)

2 cups marinara sauce (sugar-free)

2 tablespoons olive oil

1 clove garlic (minced)

Salt and pepper to taste

Fresh basil for garnish

**Preparation Method:**

Preheat the oven to 400 degrees Fahrenheit.

Season the spaghetti squash halves with salt and pepper and drizzle with olive oil.

Place the squash on a baking pan and cut side down.

Roast for 35-40 minutes, or until the potatoes are fork-tender.

Scrape out the spaghetti squash strands with a fork.

In a saucepan, heat the marinara sauce with the minced garlic.

Garnish with fresh basil and serve the sauce over the spaghetti squash strands.

Nutritional Information (per serving):

Calories: 140

Carbs: 25g

Protein: 2g

Fat: 5g

Fiber: 6g

Sugar: 8g

## Turkey Meatball Soup

Prep Time: 20 minutes

Cook Time: 30 minutes

Servings: 6

**Ingredients:**

1 lb ground turkey

6 cups chicken broth (low sodium)

2 carrots (sliced)

2 celery stalks (sliced)

1 onion (diced)

2 cloves garlic (minced)

1 tablespoon olive oil

Salt and pepper to taste

1 teaspoon dried oregano

**Preparation Method:**

To make meatballs, combine the ground turkey, salt, pepper, and oregano in a mixing bowl.

Heat olive oil in a big pot and sauté onions and garlic until transparent.

Cook for a few minutes more after adding the carrots and celery.

Bring the chicken broth to a boil.

Cook for 20 minutes after gently dropping the meatballs into the simmering stock.

Serve immediately.

Nutritional Information (per serving):

Calories: 190

Carbs: 10g

Protein: 18g

Fat: 8g

Fiber: 2g

Sugar: 3g

## Roasted Chicken with Brussel Sprouts

Prep Time: 15 minutes

Cook Time: 40 minutes

Servings: 4

**Ingredients:**

4 chicken thighs

2 cups Brussel sprouts (halved)

2 tablespoons olive oil

Salt and pepper to taste

2 cloves garlic (minced)

1 tablespoon rosemary (chopped)

**Preparation Method:**

Preheat the oven to 425°F/220°C.

Toss Brussel sprouts with olive oil, garlic, salt, pepper, and rosemary in a mixing bowl.

Season the chicken thighs with salt & pepper and place them on a baking pan.

Distribute the Brussel sprouts around the chicken.

Roast for 35-40 minutes, or until the chicken is done and the brussel sprouts are caramelized.

Serve immediately.

Nutritional Information (per serving):

Calories: 280

Carbs: 8g

Protein: 22g

Fat: 18g

Fiber: 3g

Sugar: 2g

## Eggplant Parmesan

Prep Time: 20 minutes

Cook Time: 40 minutes

Servings: 4

**Ingredients:**

1 large eggplant (sliced)

1 cup almond flour

1 cup marinara sauce (sugar-free)

1 cup mozzarella cheese (shredded)

¼cup parmesan cheese (grated)

2 eggs (beaten)

1 teaspoon dried oregano

Salt and pepper to taste

Olive oil for frying

**Preparation Method:**

Dip each eggplant slice in beaten eggs, then in almond flour seasoned with salt, pepper, and oregano.

Heat the olive oil in a skillet. Fry the eggplant slices on each sides till golden brown.

Preheat the oven to 375 degrees Fahrenheit.

Layer the fried eggplant slices, marinara sauce, and cheeses in a baking dish.

Repeat the layers until all of the ingredients have been utilized, concluding with a cheese layer on top.

Bake for 20 minutes, or until the cheese melts and becomes bubbly.

Serve immediately.

Nutritional Information (per serving):

Calories: 310

Carbs: 15g

 Protein: 15g

Fat: 22g

Fiber: 6g

Sugar: 6g

## Cabbage and Beef Stew

Prep Time: 15 minutes

Cook Time: 45 minutes

Servings: 6

**Ingredients:**

1 lb ground beef

4 cups cabbage (chopped)

1 can (14 oz) diced tomatoes

1 onion (diced)

2 cloves garlic (minced)

6 cups beef broth (low sodium)

2 tablespoons olive oil

Salt and pepper to taste

**Preparation Method:**

Heat the olive oil in a big pot.

Sauté the onions and garlic until transparent.

Cook until the ground meat is browned.

Pour in the beef broth, diced tomatoes, and cabbage, if using.

Bring to a boil and reduce to a low heat and also cook for 30 minutes.

Season with salt and pepper and serve.

Nutritional Information (per serving):

Calories: 220

Carbs: 10g

Protein: 18g

Fat: 12g

Fiber: 3g

Sugar: 5g

## Shrimp and Broccoli Stir-Fry

Prep Time: 15 minutes

Cook Time: 10 minutes

Servings: 4

**Ingredients:**

1 lb shrimp (peeled and deveined)

2 cups broccoli florets

2 tablespoons soy sauce (low sodium)

1 tablespoon olive oil

2 cloves garlic (minced)

1 teaspoon ginger (grated)

1 tablespoon sesame seeds

**Preparation Method:**

 Heat the olive oil in a skillet.

Sauté the garlic and ginger until fragrant.

Stir in the broccoli for 3 minutes.

Cook the prawns until they turn pink.

Toss in the soy sauce to coat evenly.

Serve garnished with sesame seeds.

Nutritional Information (per serving):

Calories: 180

Carbs: 6g

Protein: 25g

Fat: 6g

Fiber: 2g

Sugar: 2g

Lentil and Spinach Curry

Prep Time: 15 minutes

Cook Time: 35 minutes

Servings: 6

**Ingredients:**

1 cup dried lentils (rinsed)

2 cups spinach (chopped)

1 can (14 oz) coconut milk

2 tablespoons curry powder

1 onion (diced)

2 cloves garlic (minced)

2 tablespoons olive oil

Salt and pepper to taste

**Preparation Method:**

In a large pot, heat the olive oil.

Sauté the onions and garlic until transparent.

Stir in the curry powder thoroughly.

Bring to a simmer with the coconut milk.

Cook for 20 minutes after adding the lentils.

When the lentils are tender, add the spinach and heat until wilted.

Season with salt and pepper before serving.

Nutritional Information (per serving):

Calories: 250

Carbs: 25g

Protein: 10g

Fat: 14g

Fiber: 10g

Sugar: 3g

# CHAPTER 5
# SNACKS

## Almond Butter Celery Sticks

Prep Time: 5 minutes

Servings: 2

**Ingredients:**

4 celery sticks, washed and trimmed

4 tablespoons almond butter (unsweetened)

**Preparation Method:**

The celery sticks should be washed and dried.

Spread a spoonful of almond butter into each celery stick groove.

Serve right away.

Nutritional Information (per serving):

Calories: 100

Carbs: 4g

Protein: 3g

Fat: 8g

Fiber: 2g

## Cottage Cheese and Cherry Tomatoes

Prep Time: 5 minutes

Servings: 2

**Ingredients:**

1 cup cottage cheese (low-fat)

10 cherry tomatoes, halved

**Preparation Method:**

Fill each serving bowl halfway with cottage cheese.

Serve with the halved cherry tomatoes on top.

Chill before serving.

Nutritional Information (per serving):

Calories: 90

Carbs: 5g

Protein: 12g

Fat: 2g

Fiber: 1g

## Roasted Chickpeas

Prep Time: 10 minutes (plus 30 minutes roasting)

Servings: 4

**Ingredients:**

2 cups chickpeas (canned, drained and rinsed)

1 tablespoon olive oil

½ teaspoon sea salt

½ teaspoon smoked paprika

**Preparation Method:**

Preheat the oven to 400 degrees Fahrenheit.

Combine chickpeas, olive oil, sea salt, and smoked paprika in a mixing bowl. Stir the chickpeas until they are well coated.

On a baking sheet, spread the chickpeas in a single layer.

Roast for 30 minutes, tossing periodically, or until crispy.

Remove from the oven and let it cool.

Nutritional Information (per serving):

Calories: 145

Carbs: 20g

Protein: 7g

Fat: 5g

Fiber: 6g

## Chia Seed and Berry Parfait

Prep Time: 10 minutes (plus a few hours or overnight for soaking)

Servings: 2

**Ingredients:**

4 tablespoons chia seeds

1 cup almond milk (unsweetened)

1 cup mixed berries (e.g., blueberries, raspberries, strawberries)

1 teaspoon vanilla extract

**Preparation Method:**

In a mixing dish, combine chia seeds, almond milk, and vanilla extract. Stir thoroughly.

Refrigerate the mixture for several hours or overnight, until it hardens to a gel-like consistency.

In a glass or container, layer chia pudding with mixed berries.

Chill before serving.

Nutritional Information (per serving):

Calories: 150

Carbs: 18g

Protein: 5g

Fat: 7g

Fiber: 8g

## Mixed Nuts and Seeds

Prep Time: 2 minutes

Servings: 2

**Ingredients:**

½ cup mixed nuts (e.g., almonds, walnuts, cashews)

2 tablespoons mixed seeds (e.g., sunflower seeds, pumpkin seeds)

**Preparation Method:**

Combine the nuts and seeds in a mixing dish.

Divide the mixture between two serving bowls or snack bags.

Nutritional Information (per serving):

Calories: 220

Carbs: 7g

Protein: 7g

Fat: 19g

Fiber: 3g

## Greek Yogurt with Cinnamon and Walnuts

Prep Time: 5 minutes

Servings: 2

**Ingredients:**

1 cup Greek yogurt (unsweetened, low-fat)

½ teaspoon cinnamon

¼cup walnuts, chopped

**Preparation Method:**

Separate the Greek yogurt into two dishes.

Sprinkle cinnamon and walnuts over each serving.

Serve with a gentle stir.

Nutritional Information (per serving):

Calories: 120

Carbs: 7g

Protein: 12g

Fat: 6g

Fiber: 1g

## Sliced Cucumber with Hummus

Prep Time: 5 minutes

Servings: 2

**Ingredients:**

1 large cucumber, sliced

½ cup hummus

**Preparation Method:**

Slice the cucumber into rounds or sticks.

Serve with hummus as a dip.

Nutritional Information (per serving):

Calories: 150

Carbs: 20g

Protein: 5g

Fat: 7g

Fiber: 5g



## Avocado and Tuna Salad

Prep Time: 10 minutes

Servings: 2

**Ingredients:**

1 ripe avocado, halved and pitted

1 can (5 oz) tuna, drained

1 tablespoon olive oil

1 tablespoon lemon juice

Salt and pepper, to taste

**Preparation Method:**

In a bowl, flake the tuna and mix with olive oil, lemon juice, salt, and pepper.

Fill in the avocado halves with the tuna mixture.

Serve immediately.

Nutritional Information (per serving):

Calories: 240

Carbs: 8g

Protein: 20g

Fat: 16g

Fiber: 6g

## Edamame Beans

Prep Time: 5 minutes (plus 5 minutes steaming)

Servings: 2

**Ingredients:**

1 cup edamame beans (frozen or fresh)

Pinch of sea salt

**Preparation Method:**

In a steamer, steam the edamame beans for about 5 minutes or until they are tender.

Sprinkle with a pinch of sea salt.

Serve warm.

Nutritional Information (per serving):

Calories: 100

Carbs: 8g

Protein: 8g

Fat: 4g

Fiber: 4g

## Coconut Almond Cookies

Prep Time: 15 minutes

Servings: 12 cookies

**Ingredients:**

1 cup almond flour

½ cup unsweetened shredded coconut

¼cup coconut oil, melted

2 tablespoons honey or stevia

½ teaspoon vanilla extract

¼teaspoon salt

**Preparation Method:**

Preheat the oven to 350°F  and line a baking sheet with parchment paper.

In a bowl, combine almond flour, shredded coconut, melted coconut oil, honey/stevia, vanilla extract, and salt.

Mix until a dough forms, then scoop spoonfuls onto the baking sheet.

Flatten each cookie slightly with a fork.

Bake until the edges turn golden brown.

Let cool before serving.

Nutritional Information (per serving - 1 cookie):

Calories: 110

Carbohydrates: 4g

Fiber: 2g

Sugars: 2g

Protein: 2g

## Avocado Chocolate Mousse

Prep Time: 10 minutes

Servings: 2

**Ingredients:**

2 ripe avocados

¼cup unsweetened cocoa powder

3 tablespoons honey or stevia

½ teaspoon vanilla extract

Pinch of salt

2 tablespoons unsweetened almond milk

**Preparation Method:**

Scoop the flesh of the avocados into a blender.

Add cocoa powder, honey/stevia, vanilla extract, salt, and almond milk.

Blend until smooth and creamy.

Divide into serving cups and refrigerate for at least 1 hour before serving.

Nutritional Information (per serving):

Calories: 240

Carbohydrates: 18g

Fiber: 10g

Sugars: 5g

Protein: 4g

## Baked Cinnamon Apples

Prep Time: 15 minutes

Servings: 4

**Ingredients:**

4 apples (such as Granny Smith or Honeycrisp)

1 teaspoon ground cinnamon

¼ teaspoon nutmeg

1 tablespoon honey or stevia (optional)

¼ cup chopped walnuts (optional)

**Preparation Method:**

Preheat the oven to 375°F (190°C). Core and slice the apples into thin rounds or wedges. Toss the apple slices in a bowl with cinnamon, nutmeg, and honey/stevia (if using). Place the coated apple slices in a baking dish and top with chopped walnuts (if using). Bake until the apples are tender.

Nutritional Information (per serving):

Calories: 90

Carbohydrates: 23g

Fiber: 4g

Sugars: 17g

Protein: 1g

## Vanilla Almond Pudding

Prep Time: 10 minutes

Servings: 4

**Ingredients:**

2 cups unsweetened almond milk

¼ cup almond flour

2 tablespoons honey or stevia

2 teaspoons vanilla extract

Pinch of salt

**Preparation Method:**

Whisk together almond milk, almond flour, honey/stevia, vanilla essence, and a bit of salt in a saucepan.

Stir frequently over medium heat until the mixture thickens (approximately 5-7 minutes).

Remove from the heat and set aside.

Refrigerate until firm (approximately 1-2 hours) in serving cups.

Nutritional Information (per serving):

Calories: 90

Carbohydrates: 7g

Fiber: 1g

Sugars: 4g

Protein: 2g

## Dark Chocolate Nut Clusters

Prep Time: 20 minutes

Servings: 12 clusters

**Ingredients:**

4 oz (about ½ cup) dark chocolate (70% cocoa or higher)

½ cup mixed nuts (almonds, walnuts, pecans), chopped

¼cup unsweetened dried cranberries

**Preparation Method:**

Line a baking sheet with parchment paper. Melt the dark chocolate in a double boiler or in the microwave in 20-second intervals, stirring in between. Stir in the chopped mixed nuts and dried cranberries. Drop spoonfuls of the mixture onto the prepared baking sheet to cool and harden.

Nutritional Information (per cluster):

Calories: 90

Carbohydrates: 7g

Fiber: 2g

Sugars: 4g

Protein: 2g

## Greek Yogurt and Berry Compote

Prep Time: 15 minutes

Servings: 2

**Ingredients:**

1 cup Greek yogurt (unsweetened)

1 cup mixed berries (strawberries, blueberries, raspberries)

1 tablespoon honey or stevia (optional)

1 teaspoon lemon zest (optional)

**Preparation Method:**

Combine the mixed berries, honey/stevia, and lemon zest in a small saucepan.

Cook, stirring occasionally, over low heat until the berries break down and a compote forms (approximately 5-7 minutes).

Allow to cool to room temperature.

Layer Greek yogurt and fruit compote in serving bowls.

Garnish with fresh berries if desired.

Nutritional Information (per serving):

Calories: 150

Carbohydrates: 18g

Fiber: 4g

Sugars: 11g

Protein: 12g

## Pumpkin Spice Muffins

Prep Time: 20 minutes

Servings: 12 muffins

**Ingredients:**

2 cups almond flour

½ cup canned pumpkin puree (unsweetened)

¼cup coconut flour

¼cup erythritol or stevia

2 teaspoons baking powder

1 teaspoon pumpkin spice mix

4 large eggs

¼cup unsweetened almond milk

¼cup melted coconut oil

1 teaspoon vanilla extract

**Preparation Method:**

Preheat the oven to 350°F (175°C) and prepare a muffin pan with paper liners.

Combine almond flour, coconut flour, erythritol/stevia, baking powder, and pumpkin spice mix in a mixing bowl.

In a separate mixing dish, combine the eggs, pumpkin puree, almond milk, melted coconut oil, and vanilla extract.

Mix together the wet and dry ingredients until completely blended.

Divide the batter among the muffin cups in an equal layer.

check by inserting a toothpick at the centre to know if it is done.

Allow the muffins to cool completely before serving.

Nutritional Information (per muffin):

Calories: 160

Carbohydrates: 7g

Fiber: 3g

Sugars: 1g

Protein: 6g

## Frozen Yogurt Bark with Nuts and Seeds

Prep Time: 10 minutes

Servings: 4

**Ingredients:**

2 cups Greek yogurt (unsweetened)

¼cup mixed nuts (almonds, walnuts, pistachios), chopped

2 tablespoons seeds (chia seeds, flax seeds)

2 tablespoons honey or stevia

½ teaspoon vanilla extract

**Preparation Method:**

Combine Greek yogurt, honey/stevia, and vanilla essence in a mixing dish.

Line a baking sheet with parchment paper and spread the yogurt mixture on it.

Evenly distribute the chopped nuts and seeds over the yogurt.

Freeze for at least 2 hours.

Cut into pieces to serve.

Nutritional Information (per serving):

Calories: 180

Carbohydrates: 11g

Fiber: 2g

Sugars: 7g

Protein: 11g

## Lemon Ricotta Cheesecake

Prep Time: 30 minutes

Servings: 8

**Ingredients:**

1 ½ cups ricotta cheese (low-fat)

3/4 cup almond flour

½ cup erythritol or stevia

3 large eggs

¼cup lemon juice

1 tablespoon lemon zest

1 teaspoon vanilla extract

**Preparation Method:**

Preheat the oven to 325°F (160°C) and lightly oil a pie dish.

Combine ricotta cheese, almond flour, erythritol/stevia, eggs, lemon juice, lemon zest, and vanilla essence in a mixing bowl.

Blend until smooth.

Fill the pie dish halfway with the mixture.

30–35 minutes, or until the center is set.

Allow to cool completely before serving.

Nutritional Information (per serving):

Calories: 210

Carbohydrates: 7g

Fiber: 1g

Sugars: 1g

Protein: 11g

**Day 1:**

Breakfast: Greek yogurt with berries and a sprinkle of nuts.

Snack: Carrot and cucumber sticks with hummus.

Lunch: Grilled chicken breast with quinoa and steamed broccoli.

Snack: Apple slices with almond butter.

Dinner: Baked salmon with a side of roasted Brussels sprouts and a small sweet potato.

**Day 2:**

Breakfast: Oatmeal with sliced banana and a dash of cinnamon.

Snack: A handful of mixed nuts.

Lunch: Turkey and avocado wrap with whole-grain tortilla.

Snack: Greek yogurt with a drizzle of honey.

Dinner: Stir-fried tofu with vegetables and brown rice.

**Day 3:**

Breakfast: Scrambled eggs with spinach and a side of whole-grain toast.

Snack: Cottage cheese with sliced peaches.

Lunch: Lentil soup with a mixed greens salad.

Snack: Celery sticks with peanut butter.

Dinner: Grilled shrimp with quinoa and roasted asparagus.

**Day 4:**

Breakfast: Whole-grain waffles topped with low-sugar fruit compote.

Snack: Cherry tomatoes with mozzarella cheese.

Lunch: Quinoa and black bean salad with a vinaigrette dressing.

Snack: Mixed berries.

Dinner: Baked chicken breast with steamed green beans and quinoa.

**Day 5:**

Breakfast: Smoothie with spinach, banana, almond milk, and a scoop of protein powder.

Snack: Edamame.

Lunch: Tuna salad on whole-grain crackers.

Snack: Sliced bell peppers with hummus.

Dinner: Grilled lean steak with roasted cauliflower and a side of brown rice.

**Day 6:**

Breakfast: Cottage cheese and pineapple.

Snack: Handful of almonds.

Lunch: Vegetable stir-fry with tofu and brown rice.

Snack: Sliced pear with cottage cheese.

Dinner: Baked cod with quinoa and steamed broccoli.

**Day 7:**

Breakfast: Avocado toast with a poached egg on top.

Snack: Sugar-free yogurt with a few walnuts.

Lunch: Spinach and feta stuffed chicken breast with a side salad.

Snack: Sliced cucumber with tzatziki sauce.

Dinner: Vegetable curry with chickpeas and a side of cauliflower rice.

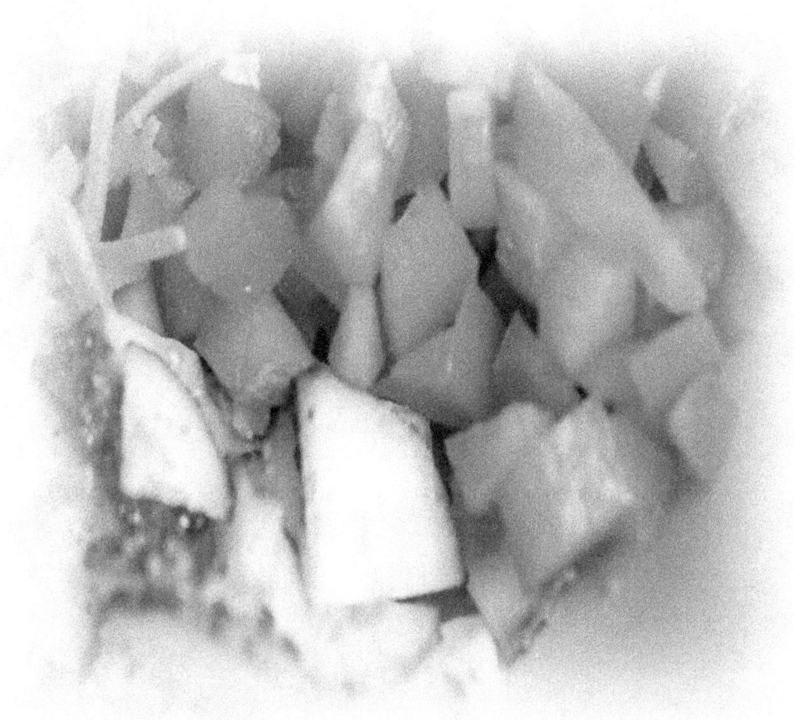

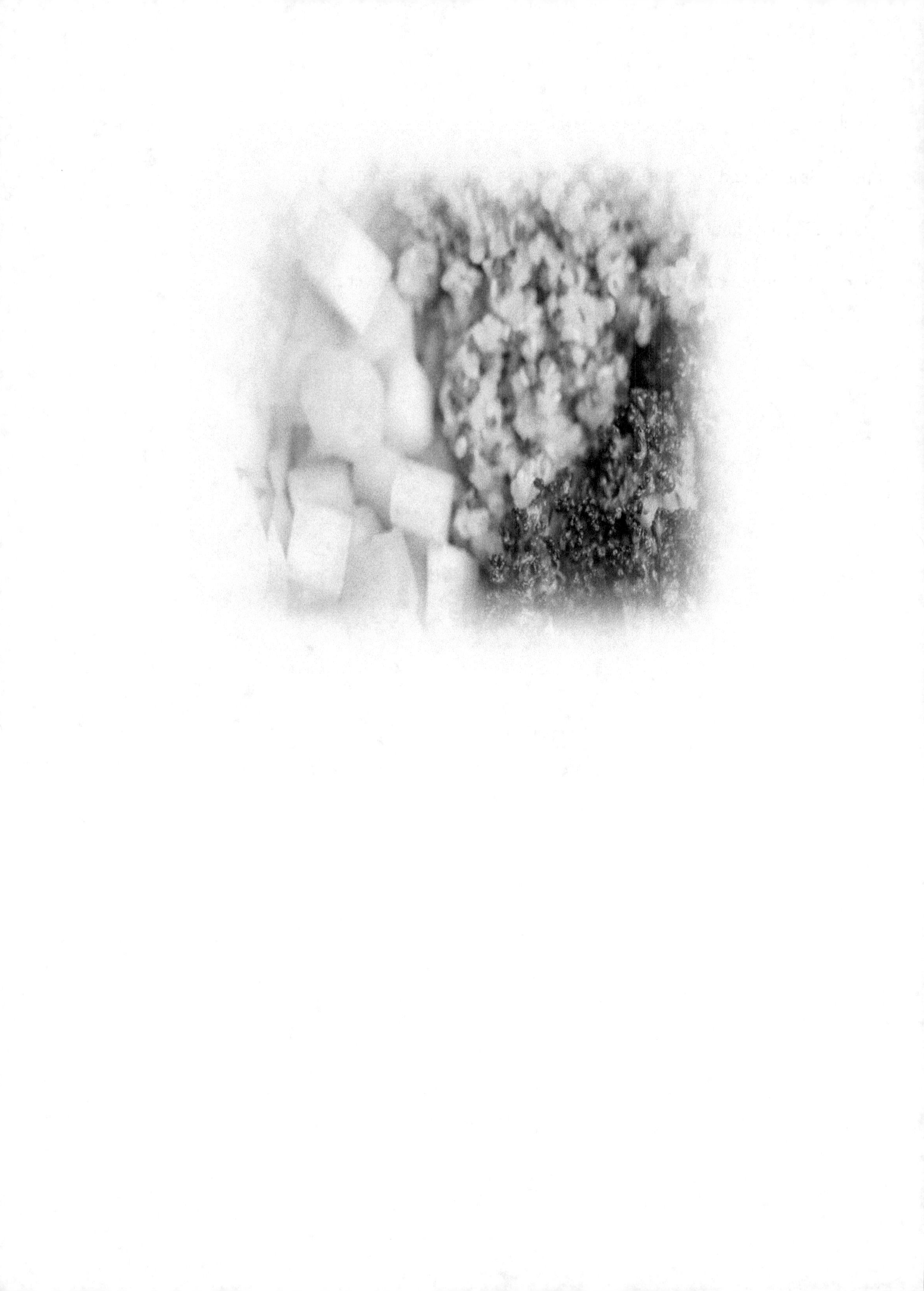

# CONCLUSION

Pre-diabetes is an important warning sign from your body that it's time to take control of your health. The good news is that you have the ability to change this condition and lower your chances of acquiring full-blown diabetes. You can take positive steps toward keeping stable blood sugar levels with a balanced diet, frequent physical activity, and the direction of healthcare specialists.

Remember that even tiny modifications in your everyday routine can have a major impact. Making healthy dietary choices, watching portion sizes, and remaining active are all important aspects of controlling pre-diabetes. It is not about deprivation, but rather about discovering delightful methods to fuel your body and prioritize your well-being.

So, don't be dismayed if you've been diagnosed with pre-diabetes. Instead, look at it as an opportunity to adopt a better, more vibrant way of life. With commitment and assistance, you can take charge of your health and lower your risk of diabetes, allowing you to live a longer, healthier, and more satisfying life.

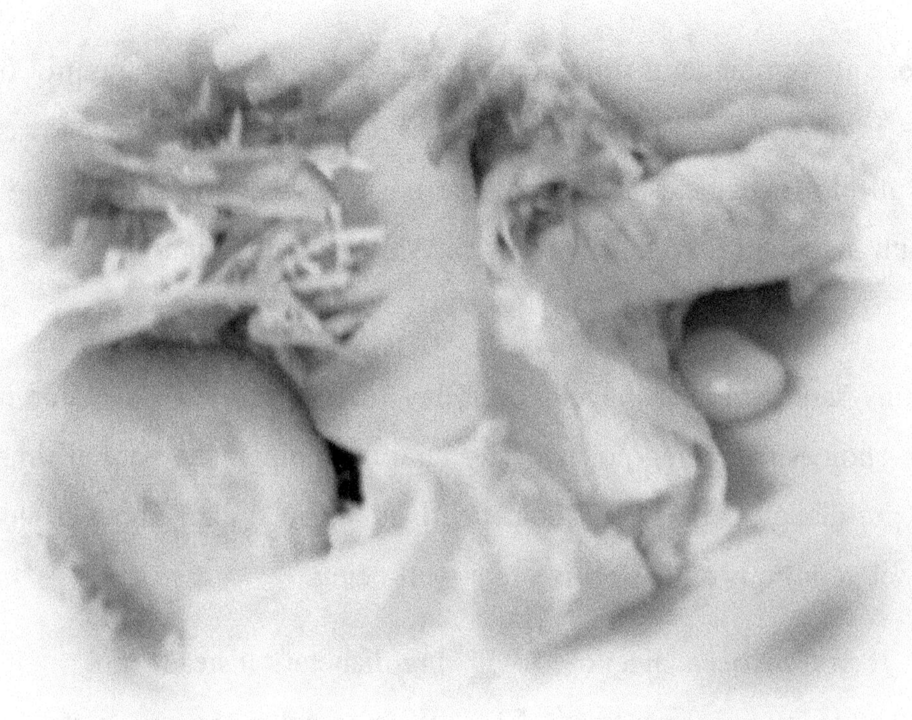